1,003
Ways to Stay Young

Other Books by Ann Hodgman

1,003 Great Things About America

1,003 Great Things About Moms

1,003 Great Things About Teachers

1,003 Great Things About Friends

1,003 Great Things About Kids

1,003 Great Things About Getting Older

1,003 Great Things to Smile About

1,003 Great Things About Being a Woman

My Baby-sitter Is a Vampire (series)

Stinky Stanley (series)

Beat This!

Beat That!

One Bite Won't Kill You

I Saw Mommy Kicking Santa Claus

1,003 Ways to Stay Young

Ann Hodgman

Andrews McMeel
Publishing, LLC

Kansas City

1,003 Ways to Stay Young

07 08 09 10 11 WKT 10 9 8 7 6 5 4 3 2

ISBN-13: 978-0-7407-5668-9

ISBN-10: 0-7407-5668-0

Library of Congress Control Number: 2006931417

1,003
Ways to Stay Young

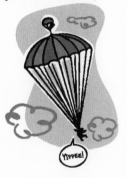

Stand up straight!

For the love of God,
trade in the minivan.

Sorry, but holding your breath
will not make you younger.

Nor will trying to erase your
wrinkles with Wite-Out.

Or vacuuming them.

You could reduce your daily intake of calories
to four hundred and live forever . . .

but it's not worth it.

"You are only young once,
and if you work it right, once is enough."
—Joe E. Lewis

Wear your hair in braids.

(With those ponytail holders that have
the colorful plastic ball on them.)

"When all else is lost, the future still remains."
—Christian Nestell Bovee

Drink through a straw.

For extra youth points: Use the straw
to blow bubbles in your drink.

For even more youth points:
The drink should be a Shirley Temple.

"Every street has two sides,
the shady side and the sunny.
When two men shake hands and part,
mark which of the two takes the sunny side;
he will be the younger man of the two."
—Edward Bulwer-Lytton

Hire a clown for your next birthday party.

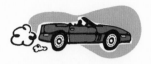

Never Admit You've
Heard Of . . .

Space Food Sticks

Rowan and Martin's Laugh-In

Platform shoes (the first time around)

Metrical

"Slicker" lip gloss

Menudo

Suzy Homemaker

The Sensuous Woman

"Mrs. Brown, You've Got a
Lovely Daughter"

"Kung-Fu Fighting"

David, Shaun, or even Patrick Cassidy

Long-playing records

Postage stamps

Rotary phones

Gasoline for under $2.50 a gallon

Extra-wide watchbands

Chuck Mangione

"The Legend of Billy Jack"

Folk-rock church services

Crispy Critters

The Hustle

"Charlie" cologne

Dippity-Doo

"In the valley of the
Jolly (ho, ho, ho) Green Giant!"

Garter belts worn "non-ironically,"
as an actual way to hold up stockings

Is going to a pediatrician at the age
of thirty-five a little much?

"I'm rubber, you're glue; everything
you say bounces off of me and
back to you" is a great retort.

For nostalgia's sake, memorize
the state capitals.

Ask your boss if spelling counts.

"The belief that youth is the happiest
time of life is founded on a fallacy.
The happiest people are those who think
the most interesting thoughts."
—William Lyon Phelps

Join a soccer team.

Or at least coach one.

Learn a magic trick.

Sign up for a life-drawing class
and blush with embarrassment.

There are some youthful habits it's good to
shed—like filing your nails in public.

Use Band-Aids with cartoon
characters on them.

Wear kneesocks or anklets with your skirts.

"Beauty is in the eye of the beholder, and it
may be necessary from time to time to give a
stupid or misinformed beholder a black eye."
—Miss Piggy

Wear mittens.

For extra youth points: Attach
your mittens to your snowsuit.

Exercise—the only real magic bullet.

Keep blabbing about how much you love whoever the flavor-of-the-month teen idol is.

"Do not commit the error common among the young, of assuming that if you cannot save the whole of mankind you have failed."
—Jan de Hartog

Ask your mom to cut your fingernails for you.

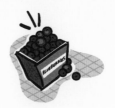

The Ten Healthiest Foods, According to the Mayo Clinic
(And One of Them Isn't Mayo!)

Apples

Almonds

Blueberries

Broccoli

Red beans

Salmon

Spinach

Sweet potatoes

Vegetable juice

Wheat germ

Eating spinach twice a week will keep your
eyesight from degenerating.

Paint the walls of your bedroom pink to give
your face a flattering youthful glow.

Take up bungee jumping, if you dare.

You could always switch from
glue back to paste.

If you dreamed of being a firefighter as a kid, join your town's volunteer firefighting crew.

Actually, do that even if you didn't dream of being a firefighter as a kid.

(The town's EMT crew could use you, too.)

"An inordinate passion for
pleasure is the secret of remaining young."
—Oscar Wilde

Remember that the future is where you're
going to spend the rest of your life.

Train your grandchildren to
call you by your first name.

Switch from edamame to Fruit Roll-Ups.

Keep your childhood teddy bear nearby . . .
if not on your bed, then on your desk.

"Seek first to understand,
then to be understood."
—Steven Covey

Dot your i's with a daisy.

We're not recommending it, but . . . would you consider a tattoo?

Bleach your teeth—easy to do, since every product on the market these days seems to contain tooth-whitener.

"You can only be young once. But you can always be immature."
—Dave Barry

Take up a new hobby, like obsessively checking for wrinkles in the mirror.

Rumor has it that adding a little fat to your diet will smooth out your skin.

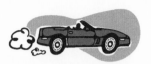

Proverbs for
Baby Boomers

An apple a day keeps the doctor away,
but an apple-cucumber mask will
tighten the skin.

Ask no questions about how others like
your cheap hair dye job, and you hear no lies
unless you run into your mother.

Beauty is only skin deep, but you have
the gallbladder of a thirty-year-old.

Blood is thicker than water,
but it would not be healthy to drink
eight glasses of blood a day.

Curiosity killed the cat, but all
that cream certainly didn't help.

Don't cut off your nose to spite your face, no matter how much you don't like that bump. (It's cute!)

Don't wash your dirty linen in public, and it's probably not a good idea to put on lipstick in front of people, either.

Every picture tells a story.
For instance, someone clearly doctored
her jowls in this one.

Fight fire with fire, but make sure
you put on some kind of mask.

Develop a taste for cotton candy.

Use "I have to do my homework"
as an excuse for getting out of stuff.

"We must always change, renew,
rejuvenate ourselves; otherwise, we harden."
—Goethe

Give your age in base fourteen.

Switch from Belgian beer to Budweiser.

"There is a fountain of youth: It is your
mind, your talents, the creativity you bring
to your life and the lives of people you love.
When you learn to tap this source,
you will truly have defeated age."
—Sophia Loren

Always carry Clearasil.

Go to a Korn concert . . .

On second thought,
that'll make you feel old.

"To stay youthful, stay useful."
—Anonymous

Must you really choose "granny glasses"
frames for your bifocals?

Throw away your flowered bathing cap.

Switch to Pluto's calendar year and you'll
instantly be 248 times younger.

"It takes a long time to learn
to become young."
—Pablo Picasso

Never use a three-way mirror again.

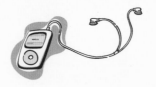

Cheer Up!
You're Still Younger Than . . .

The oldest mammal (the fin whale):
114 years old

The stuff under your son's bed:
1,003 years old

The oldest (still-living) tree:
at least 4,000 years old

That dumb joke your father always tells:
6,213 years old

The first modern human:
200,000 years old

Oldest fossil:
53.5 million years old

Your car:
4 million years old

The diamond in your diamond ring:
3.3 billion years old

The first bacteria:
3.5 billion years old

Parents of first bacteria:
3.5 billion and twenty-six years old

The earth:
4.5 billion years old

The sun:
5 billion years old

The universe:
13.7 billion years old
(or at least that's what it admits to)

The leftovers in Aunt Rita's refrigerator:
13.8 billion years old

Aunt Rita: 13.9 billion years old

They say people look immature when they chew gum—why not give it a try?

Start wearing one of those Old Navy spray colognes that smell like water instead of Grandma.

"As long as you can still be disappointed, you are still young."
—Sarah Churchill

It's never too late to start using sunscreen.

And if it *is* too late for that, it's *really*
never too late to get a peel.

Elastic-waist skirts let you dance
like a teenager!

According to Mamie Eisenhower,
lying in bed all day prevents wrinkles.

"I'll tell ya how to stay young:
Hang around with older people."
—Bob Hope

Mom was right. Eat your broccoli.

Buy a cute little sports car—after making sure
you can climb in and out of it.

"You are as young as your faith, as old
as your doubt; as young as your
self-confidence, as old as your fear; as young
as your hope, as old as your despair."
—Douglas MacArthur

Read hard, boring books so you'll
think you're still in school.

Hey, look at this cool seashell!

Send your memos in invisible ink.

(Hint: Lemon juice
makes great invisible ink.)

"I refuse to admit that I am more than fifty-two, even if that makes my children illegitimate."
—Lady Nancy Astor

For heaven's sake, stop making those little groaning sounds when you stand up or sit down.

Keep your AARP card at home.

Don't ask if there's a senior
discount on the bus.

Never admit you don't know
how to use your iPod.

"If you're looking for youth, you're looking
for longevity, just take a dose of rock 'n' roll.
It keeps you going. Just like the
caffeine in your coffee."
—Hank Ballard

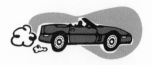

Second Acts
(And Sometimes Third and Fourth and More)

Michael Miliken: from criminal to philanthropist

David Lee Roth: from has-been rock legend to emergency medical technician to national radio talk-show host

Jesse Ventura: from professional wrestler to Minnesota governor to talk-show host to Harvard teacher

Magic Johnson: from basketball player to successful entrepreneur

Arnold Schwarzenegger: from Mr. Universe
to movie star to California governor

Arianna Huffington: from prominent
Republican to prominent Democrat to
founder of a prominent Web site

Vaclav Havel: from writer and playwright to dissident to president of Czechoslovakia

Jerry Springer: from mayor of Cincinnati to provocative TV talk-show host for hicks

Sean Diddy Combs: Puff Daddy to P Diddy to Diddy

Madonna: singer to movie star to
Kabbalist to wife and mother

John Travolta: from dancer to movie star to
"whatever-happened-to?" movie star

Pete Rose: from Cincinnati Reds baseball legend to banned gambler to potential baseball Hall of Famer to banned gambler

Brigitte Bardot: from French movie sex kitten to world-renowned animal-rights activist

Doris Day: from American movie "good clean fun sex kitten" to another world-renowned animal-rights activist

William Shakespeare:
from greatest playwright in the English language to "maybe he didn't write them all" to "yes, he probably did write them all"

No more talk about your
last will and testament!

Keep the news that you take
Lipitor to yourself.

Color your hair . . . immediately.

Remember: Wearing a veil sends
the wrong message.

"Anyone who stops learning is old, whether
this happens at twenty or eight. Anyone
who keeps on learning not only remains
young, but becomes constantly more valuable
regardless of physical capacity."
—Harvey Ullman

Exfoliate, exfoliate, exfoliate.

And then exfoliate some more.

Somehow, track down the fountain of youth.

(And while you're at it, build a time machine.)

"If you want to recapture your youth,
just cut off his allowance."
—Al Bernstein

Move to Canada, where you can buy
prescription-strength hydroquinone
(age-spot fader) over the counter.

Actually read your computer manual,
so that you can actually learn how your
computer works.

Comfortable shoes will make you happier, and being happier will reduce stress, and reducing stress will make you younger.

Unless you're the type who feels sexy in stiletto heels. If so, go for it!

Take up your childhood dream of inventing something that will make you rich.

(And thinking up inventions works better
than counting sheep at night.)

"To find joy in work is to discover the
fountain of youth."
—Pearl S. Buck

Don't over-pluck your eyebrows.
After awhile they won't grow back.

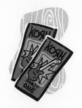

Believe It or Not, Some People Would *Like* to Be Older . . .

One day old: If only I'd been born forty-eight hours ago instead of twenty-four, they'd let me go home with my parents.

One week old: If only I were two weeks old, my "startle" reflex wouldn't be so hair-trigger.

Two weeks old: When will I be
four weeks old so I can start smiling?

Four weeks old: Maybe by the time
I'm two months old, I'll be sleeping
through the damn night.

Two months old: I'm so tired of staying
where they put me. Just one more month
and I'll be able to roll over . . .

Three months old: Rolling over is boring.
I wish I were six months old so I could sit up.

Ten months old: If only I were one, I could
walk instead of this stupid crawling.

One year old: If only I were eighteen months
old, they'd call me a toddler instead of a baby.

Eighteen months old: When I'm two, I'll be able to talk instead of this babbling.

Two years old: If only I were three, I'd be over the terrible twos.

Three years old: Pre-K 3 sounds so . . . young compared to Pre-K 4!

Four years old: If only
I were in kindergarten!

Five years old: When I'm six, I'll be
able to read real words instead of just
learning the dumb alphabet.

Six years old: If only I were seven, I'd be able to read everything without having someone tell me, "Sound it out!"

Seven years old: If only I could play in the eight-and-over soccer league!

Eight years old: The great thing about turning nine is that I'll be able to say "I'm almost ten."

Nine years old: When I'm ten, I'll be one-tenth of a century old.

Ten years old: If only I were eleven,
I wouldn't have a zero in my age.

Eleven years old: Twelve sounds so much
cooler—you're a real preteen then.

Twelve years old: Thirteen-year-olds
get invited to all the bat mitzvah and
bar mitzvah parties.

Thirteen years old: I can't wait to be fourteen and be in high school.

Fourteen years old: If only I were fifteen, I could have a *quinceañera*, if we were Hispanic.

Fifteen years old: When I'm sixteen, I'll be able to drive to school instead of going on the bus with all the losers and babies.

Sixteen years old: If only I were sixteen and a half, I'd be allowed to drive my friends to school too.

Seventeen years old: If only I were eighteen, I'd be able to vote and get the drinking law changed back to eighteen.

Eighteen years old: At least when you're nineteen, you don't seem like a teenager anymore.

Nineteen years old: If only I were twenty, people would stop calling me a "girl."

Twenty years old: When the hell am I going to be legal?

Twenty-one years old: If only I were twenty-two, I'd be able to stop going to all these bars just to prove that I can.

Twenty-two-years old: I hope that when I'm thirty I'll have all this career stuff sorted out.

Thirty years old: If only I were forty, I'd have all this start-a-family stuff sorted out.

Thirty-nine years old: At least when I'm forty, people won't think I'm lying about my age the way they do now.

Fifty years old: When I get to sixty, maybe I'll have all this "middle age" stuff sorted out.

Sixty years old: If only I were sixty-five, I could retire.

Sixty-five years old: If only I were seventy, I could retire.

Seventy years old: If only I were eighty,
I could retire.

Eighty years old: Maybe by ninety
I'll have that "serene resignation" they
always talk about.

Ninety years old: At least you get a letter from the president when you turn one hundred.

One hundred years old:
From here on in, every year brings me closer to a world record.

Wearing sunglasses protects your eyes just as
wearing sunscreen protects your skin.

They say frowning causes wrinkles.

To be on the safe side, maybe you should give
up all facial expressions.

"I won't grow up,
I don't want to wear a tie.
And a serious expression in
the middle of July . . . "
—Carolyn Leigh

Learn to dance—any style you want.

(But don't let anyone take your picture while
you're dancing.)

Adopt a kitten.

"One of the delights known to age,
and beyond the grasp of youth,
is that of Not Going."
—Anthony Burgess

Plant a garden.

Or even just a tomato plant in a pot.

Don't be afraid of teenagers on the sidewalk.
They're not thinking about you.

"There is a way to look at the past.
Don't hide from it. It will not catch
you—if you don't repeat it."
—Pearl Bailey

Take time to play. (Note: Watching tennis on
TV does not count as "playing.")

Eat plenty of blueberries and other brightly colored fruits that are rich in antioxidants.

Shave your legs every day.
Men shave daily; why not you?

Use conditioner as shaving cream.

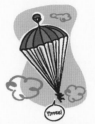

Good vs. Bad

A spring in your step is good . . .

Skipping everywhere you go is ludicrous.

A smile on your face is good . . .

Constant, meaningless laughter is annoying.

Taking up pole-vaulting is good . . .

Going around on a pogo stick
is just plain silly.

Using concealer under your eyes is good . . .

Wearing a Lindsay Lohan mask is crazy.

Using a loofah on your dry legs is good . . .

Getting a leg peel is extreme.

Auditing a college course is good . . .

Attending an all-night kegger is moronic.

Broadening your interests is good . . .

Learning taxidermy is creepy.

Boogie-boarding is good . . .

Shuffleboard is a no-no.

A subscription to *Entertainment Weekly* is good . . .

A subscription to *Highlights* is even better . . .

A subscription to *Osteoporosis Oracle* is out of the question.

"Much education today is monumentally ineffective. All too often we are giving young people cut flowers when we should be teaching them to grow their own plants."
—John Gardner

Take a multivitamin, even if science proves that they're useless.

Spend more time with kids—your own or someone else's.

"It is better to waste one's youth
than to do nothing with it at all."
—Georges Courteline

Reread all your best self-help books.

And all your favorite children's books.

Start wearing a new color. (Hint: not black.)

"Don't waste your youth growing up."
—Anonymous

"To get back one's youth, one
merely has to repeat one's follies."
—Oscar Wilde

It's never too late to eat more fiber!

Figure out what you've always
wanted to do—and do it.

Memorize an interesting new fact daily.

"Maturity is often more absurd than youth
and very frequently is most unjust to youth."
—Thomas A. Edison

Stay abreast of current events.

(Which does not mean
complaining about them.)

Never assume that just because you're getting older, the world is going downhill.

"To get back to my youth,
I would do anything except take exercise,
get up early, or be respectable."
—Oscar Wilde

Attack those cluttered closets. It won't make you younger, but believe us—everyone is talking about what a mess your closets are.

Don't be scared to swim in cold water.
It always feels better once your head is under.

🕯

And don't just sit on the beach reading. Build
a sandcastle or take a walk or something.

🕯

"I live in that solitude which is painful in
youth, but delicious in the years of maturity."
—Albert Einstein

If you drink hard liquor,
switch to wine or beer.

If you drink regular soft drinks,
switch to diet ones.

Better yet, switch to seltzer.

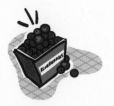

Old, Out-of-Date
Foods to Avoid

Melba toast

Nilla wafers

Cottage cheese with canned peaches

Saltines

Oyster crackers

Minute Rice

Anything served in a patty shell

Anything served on toast

Rice pudding

Harvey's Bristol Cream

Tapioca

Fig Newtons

Aspic

Molded salad

Jell-O

Sherbet

Horehound drops

Sourballs

Poached eggs

Fruit cup

Prune juice

Beef bouillon

Poached chicken

"In youth we learn; in age we understand."
—Marie von Ebner-Eschenbach

Protest injustice.

Challenge your assumptions.

Purge the words "When I was your age . . . "
from your lexicon.

Remember: If you've thought something before, you've probably said it before, too.

Keep on top of your weeding, or your house will start to look haunted.

Give out good candy at Halloween—not cough drops or mints or stuff like that.

"Youth is largely a habit. So is romance. . . .
Both habits may be prolonged far beyond the
moping limits of custom, and need never be
abandoned unless we become sincerely and
unregretfully tired of them."
—Richard Le Gallienne

Make sure to vote, even if it's raining.

Try not to serve leftover Meals on
Wheels at dinner parties.

Never say that the *New Yorker* cartoons used to be funnier in your day.

"Youth smiles without any reason.
It is one of its chiefest charms."
—Thomas Gray

Pinching a child's cheek is a great way to be mistaken for a witch.

"When in doubt, throw it out."
—Peg Bracken

Try to resist the Early Bird Special.

And easy-listening radio.

And fumbling for the correct change.

"I mention my age because I find people in this country—women, not men, of course—women are so troubled by their age. There's a culture of youth, and it's a phony culture."
—Teresa Heinz Kerry

Master the art of French cooking.

Party a little less hearty.

A sports deodorant may
make you feel sportier.

Take a personal day for no reason.

"The secret of eternal youth
is arrested development."
—Alice Roosevelt Longworth

Stairs are better than elevators.

Don't stash tissues up your sleeve.
Throw them out like a normal person.

Might as well give Restylane a try . . .

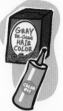

Mother Goose
Stays Young

Hickory dickory dock,
Time's running out on your clock . . .

Jack and Jill ran up the hill
To blast their glutes like iron . . .

A-tisket, a-tasket,
Put Centrum in your basket . . .

Twinkle, twinkle, little star
Don't need reading glasses to
know what you are!

Mary's little lamb followed her to
extension classes one night . . .

The eency-weency spider vein
Climbed up her leg one day and the
next day, she went to the dermatologist
to have it removed.

The farmer in the dell, the farmer in the dell,
The farmer takes a trophy wife . . .

Hot cross buns,
Hot cross buns,
Don't worry. The surgeon can take care of it.

Humpty Dumpty sat on a wall,
Humpty Dumpty had a great fall,
And now Humpty has to have a
hip replacement.

Jack be nimble,
Jack be quick,
Doesn't Jack look good for eighty-three?!

Jack Sprat could eat no fat,
His wife could eat no lean,
And yet, they both had good cholesterol!

This old man, he played one,
Uh-oh, time for the home!

"Youth condemns; maturity condones."
—Amy Lowell

Carry your own luggage—it will
make you stronger.

Isn't it about time you got
that graduate degree?

Learn to use chopsticks if you
don't already know.

Take a "service vacation."

"Old age has its pleasures, which,
though different, are not less than
the pleasures of youth."
—W. Somerset Maugham

Never say that today's music is just noise.

Or that the culture is in decline.

Go to a horror movie—and scream
as loud as you want.

And as long as you're shaking yourself up,
how about a roller coaster?

And parasailing?

And hang gliding?

"Creativity is not merely the innocent
spontaneity of our youth and childhood;
it must also be married to the passion
of the adult human being, which is a passion
to live beyond one's death."
—Rollo May

Volunteer to be a kid's mentor.

Don't become timid.

And don't dither.

Or fret.

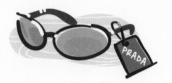

Hang on to These,
No Matter How Old You Get!

Blue jeans
(So what if they have an elastic waist?)

Sneakers

Fisherman's sweaters

Jelly beans

Bathing

Giggling at inappropriate moments

Catching snowflakes on your tongue

Sitting on the floor sometimes

Having a favorite baseball team

Rock 'n' roll

Listening to your Rice Krispies
when you pour in the milk

Your love of John Cusack

Crying at sentimental TV commercials

Your dreams of being a poet

Cutting your toenails

"Time, still as he flies, adds increase
to her truth, and gives to her mind
what he steals from her youth."
—Edward Moore

Do something that will really get
you talked about.

Don't drive down the middle of the road,
either literally or figuratively.

Go ahead—treat yourself to cotton candy.

Resign your cushy job on principle.

"Prove that you understand the worth of time
by employing it well. Then youth will be
delightful, old age will bring few regrets, and
life will become a beautiful success."
—Louisa May Alcott

Don't make yourself a martyr to your kids.
(Is the neck really your favorite
piece of chicken?)

Take note of pantyhose trends. Nothing
looks more dated than "suntan" when "nude"
is the prevailing color.

That "when I am an old woman, I shall wear
purple" thing . . . maybe not.

But red eyeglasses are good.

"Character contributes to beauty.
It fortifies a woman as her youth fades. A
mode of conduct, a standard of courage,
discipline, fortitude, and integrity can do a
great deal to make a woman beautiful."
—Jacqueline Bisset

Once a week, send an appreciative
postcard to someone.

Don't let the dust settle.

Rest for twenty minutes with avocado slices
under your eyes to relieve puffiness.

(Eye puffiness, that is. Avocado slices
on your stomach won't do much.)

"What's a man's age? He must hurry
more, that's all; Cram in a day, what
his youth took a year to hold."
—Robert Browning

Think of yourself as "mature"
rather than "old."

Drink as much coffee as you want.
It doesn't seem to hurt anything.

Take up mountain biking.
Everyone else your age is doing it.

"Education is the best friend. An educated
person is respected everywhere. Education
beats the beauty and the youth."
—Chanakya

Don't put off that bunionectomy any longer.

Learn not to interrupt.
It makes you seem deaf.

When people ask how you are, just say
"Fine, thanks. How are you?" Don't give them
the whole song and dance.

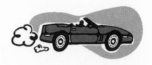

Things You Should Maybe

Let Go of After Forty
(No Matter How Young
They Make You Feel)

Your security blanket

Your "My Little Pony" collection
in the living room

Your dreams of being a rock star
The diamond-and-platinum
"grill" on your teeth

Black nail polish

Black fishnets

Plunging necklines

Screaming when you see a spider

Overalls, unless you're a farmer

MySpace.com

Waist-length blond hair

The word "awesome"

Lollipops in public

Plastic "safety" scissors

A visible belly button

Crucifixes as a fashion statement

Your tricycle

Your pacifier

"All those things you fought
against as a youth: You begin to realize they're
stereotypes because they're true."
—David Cronenberg

Stop sweating the small stuff, like the fact that
squirrels keep robbing your bird feeder.

Never let yourself be seen at any
slot machines anywhere.

"If wisdom's ways you wisely seek,
five things observe with care: to whom
you speak, of whom you speak, and how,
and when, and where."
—Caroline Ingalls

Facial exercises really work!

No one can see your wrinkles if you
keep the lights off and the shades
down and a bag over your head.

Maybe you can get California Closets
to declutter your brain, too.

"If we keep well and cheerful, we
are always young and at last die in youth even
when in years would count as old."
—Tryon Edwards

Never say, "I feel a draft."

Not that it will exactly keep you young, but isn't it about time you learned to read a map?

Remember: When the "Don't Walk" sign is flashing, it's OK to cross the street if no cars are coming.

"At times it seems that I am living my life backward, and that at the approach of old age my real youth will begin."
—André Gide

Bring something interesting to read at the doctor's office, instead of uselessly fretting about how long you have to wait.

You don't have to embrace pop culture, but you shouldn't shun it.

Get the kind of cough drops that don't have crinkly-sounding wrappers.

You never need to outgrow Elmo
from *Sesame Street*.

"Trivia is a game played by those
who realize that they have misspent their
youth but do not want to let go of it."
—Edwin Goodgold

Stash pairs of reading glasses
everywhere so no one will ever hear you say,
"Where did I leave my glasses?"

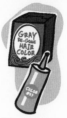

How to Tell When You've Had Too Much Plastic Surgery

Your eyebrows are concealed by your hairline.

Your smile is twelve inches long.

A little boy thinks your head is a jack-o'-lantern.

A little girl says, "Mommy, why is that lady surprised?"

You can't close your eyes all the way.

"Bee-stung" doesn't come *close* to describing your lips.

Neither does "trout pout."

You can't sit down because of
your butt implants.

You can't stand up straight because
of your thigh lift.

Your nostrils are wide enough
to hold marshmallows.

Squirrels keep scrabbling at your face
because they think you've got walnuts
stuffed into your cheekbones.

Your neck is so tight that you can't
turn your head.

Everyone tells you your ponytail is too tight,
and you're not wearing a ponytail.

People keep saying, "Joan Rivers!
Can I have your autograph?"

Michael Jackson calls you for advice.

You can bounce a dime off your cheek.

Your breasts point straight toward the
ceiling when you lie on your back.

On Halloween, people ask,
"And who are you supposed to be?"

Your photo turns up on
www.awfulplasticsurgery.com.

Resist the urge to show people
pictures of your grandchildren.

"Attitude is a little thing that
makes a big difference."
—Winston Churchill

Go ahead and splurge on sheets.

Work on your stretches while you watch TV.

And do some crunches, while you're at it.

And practice balancing on one foot at a time.

"We either make ourselves miserable, or happy
and strong. The amount of work is the same."
—Francesca Reigler

Limber up your brain by memorizing
a poem every week.

Always mute the commercials—
it reduces stress.

Clear your conscience by apologizing
to someone who deserves it.

(Come on—you know a name popped into
your head when you read that.)

"Youth is the gift of nature, but age
is a work of art."
—Stanislaw Lec

It's never too late to take up meditating.

Really brush the way the dentist says, instead
of doing it the way you've done it all your life.

Step splashily into puddles,
instead of avoiding them.

"You cannot control what happens
to you, but you can control your attitude
toward what happens to you, and in that,
you will be mastering change rather than
allowing it to master you."
—Brian Tracy

Never say, "I only watch PBS."

Never say, "I only listen to NPR."

Start using a new spice when you cook.

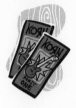

What Doesn't Work

Hot pants

The magic beans that elf gave you yesterday

The Cabbage Soup Diet

Frownies and Wrinkies

Gravity-inversion systems

Sleeping on your back

"Mink Oil"

Dressing like a preteen

Singing along with your headphones
on the subway

Wishing upon a star

"The more expensive the moisturizer,
the better!"

Bathing in milk

Immersing your face in ice because
Paul Newman says it works for him

Wearing your old go-go boots

Treating your kids like pals

♫

Human growth hormone

♫

Pulling your belt way up over your gut
(or letting it hang below)

Letting your thong show

Piercing your eyebrow

Sunbathing

Marrying a trophy spouse

Calling all your friends "Grandma"

Deciding not to celebrate your birthday

Switching your birthday to February 29

"Years wrinkle the skin, but to give up
enthusiasm wrinkles the soul."
—Douglas MacArthur

Subscribe to a magazine with the exact
opposite philosophy of yours.

Visit a place you've never wanted to see.

Then, to reward yourself, visit a place
you've always wanted to see.

"Coast and you will go downhill."
—Dave Roberson,
former New Trier swim coach

If you have no time to exercise,
at least do a few push-ups.

Stand in front of the mirror and let your
stomach all the way out. Then suck it in.
What an improvement!

Go on—give the monkey bars a try again.

"There is always some specific moment when
we become aware that our youth is gone; but,
years after, we know it was much later."
—Mignon McLaughlin

Lose the long gray ponytail if you're a guy.

(And also if you're a gal.)

"Use what talents you possess: The woods would be very silent if no birds sang there except those that sang the best."
—Henry Van Dyke

Become a nun. They don't care
about stuff like staying young.

Have a parent-mandated bedtime.

Skipping is good aerobic exercise, besides
being ridiculously young-looking.

"Forget your experiences, grab the lessons,
and keep on swinging!"
—Errol Smith

It's never too late to start watching
The Simpsons.

Keep your nails blunt instead of pointy.

And no red nail polish!

"Take a course in good water and air;
and in the eternal youth of Nature you
may renew your own. Go quietly, alone;
no harm will befall you."
—John Muir

One color you never see on actual young
people: ash blonde.

Buy an incubator and hatch some quail eggs.
It won't make you younger, but haven't you
always wanted to try it?

"Be master of your petty annoyances and
conserve your energies for the big, worthwhile
things. It isn't the mountain ahead that wears
you out—it's the grain of sand in your shoe."
—Robert Service

Penny loafers always look younger
with pennies in them.

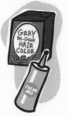

Lipstick Colors
to Steer Clear Of

Rosacea

"Old As the Earth" Terra-cotta

Rusty Copper

Very Old Wine

The Bloom Is off the Rose

Spawning Salmon

Summer's End Geranium

Retirement Red

Chestnut

Waxen Lilies

Hemoglobin

Fall Foliage

Wilted Gardenia

Bloodshot

Dusk

Vintage

Buy yourself a big red balloon.

Then let go of the string and cry as the balloon floats away.

"Yes, the experience of all stages
of life are valuable, not just of youth."
—Daniel Petrie

Resolve not to die until you've learned
to give a speech in public.

And also not until you've found
the perfect fried chicken.

"Hope is a light diet, but very stimulating."
—Balzac

Go camping. You'll feel so great when you can
sleep in your own bed again!

If you trip and fall in front of a lot of people,
laugh instead of suing.

"Youth has no age."
—Pablo Picasso

You'd get a better perspective if you
climbed a tree once in awhile.

Make sure your next hobby involves
being outside in some way.

"The willow which bends to the tempest often
escapes better than the oak which resists it."
—Sir Walter Scott

Start putting "Miss" and "Mrs." in
front of all your friends' names.

Start refusing to eat peas because "someone
at school told me they're poison."

Don't just lie about your age.
Lie about your parents' ages, too.

"He who is of calm and happy
nature will hardly feel the pressure of age,
but to him who is of an opposite disposition
youth and age are equally a burden."
—Plato

Switch from boring showers to
fun bubble baths.

Stop using a purse; start using
a messenger bag.

Whenever you get tired of walking, whine that you want someone to carry you.

"There are three periods in life: youth, middle age, and 'how well you look.'"
—Nelson Rockefeller

An apple a day has to do something or other besides just keeping the doctor away.

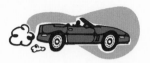

Words to Avoid When
You Place That Personals Ad

Spry

Well preserved

Spunky

Circling the drain

Arthritic

Sage

Ashen

Hobbling

Furrowed

Alert

Not over the hill yet

Full of wisdom

Slightly shriveled

Forgetful

A bit crotchety

Totally gray

Curmudgeonly

Monied

Depression baby

A faceful of laugh lines

A character

Codger

Stately

Not demented

Of a certain age

All there

Lively

Full of life

Still kicking

Senior

Eccentric

Old dear

Old

Gnarled

Ambulatory

At peace

Kids eat a lot of ice cream, and look how young they are!

Watch *The Wizard of Oz* once a year, the way you did when you were little.

"Keep true to the dreams of your youth."
—Friedrich von Schiller

Great news! Many kinds of stress protect us from Alzheimer's, arthritis, and heart disease.

More great news! Subjecting cells to moderate stress can have beneficial cosmetic effects.

Denial.

Denial, denial, denial.

"Age has been the perfect fire
extinguisher for flaming youth."
—Navjot Singh Sidhu

Hire a pilot to take you on an
acrobatic airplane ride.

(Better yet, hire a pilot to take you to
Tahiti on a private plane.)

(Better yet, get your pilot's license.)

Somehow, have so much money that you don't care how old you are.

"It can make you sad to look at pictures from your youth. So there's a trick to it. The trick is not to look at the later pictures."
—Jerry Stiller

There are a number of promising substances on the market that can actually rejuvenate your cells, but we're not allowed to reveal their names.

Green tea really helps!

So does silymarin, which is found in the milk
thistle family—whatever that is.

They also say herbal tea may
reverse the aging process.

OK, we admit that's a stretch, but at least you
won't be up all at night.

"Invention is the talent of youth,
and judgment of age."
—Jonathan Swift

Fish oil. Why not?

Play charades at a party and you'll feel ten
years younger.

(But play Twister and you may feel ten years
older, at least the next day.)

Go on a picnic in the park.

"Youth is when you're allowed to stay up late on New Year's Eve. Middle age is when you're forced to."
—Bill Vaughan

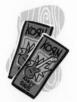

The Youngest-Sounding Things to Say on a First Date

"I'm too little to go steady."

"My parents gave me a midnight curfew."

"I hope you invite me to the prom."

"Your epidermis is showing!"

"Look up, look down, look at my thumb—
gee, you're dumb!"

"Will you test me on my words?
I have a spelling test tomorrow."

"Can't tomorrow afternoon.
I have cheerleading practice."

"I can't wait until I'm old enough to vote."

"I'll buy the beer. I have a fake ID."

"Maybe it'll be different when I'm gray, but I don't think I'll ever dye my hair."

"A lot of people my age never even heard of the Vietnam War."

"I think it must be a growing pain."

"Don't you hate going to Sweet Sixteens?"

"My pediatrician says . . ."

"Omigod. I have, like, so much of my student loan to pay off!"

"I can eat anything I want and not gain weight, but they say your metabolism changes."

"Love to, but I'm grounded."

"How much do your parents give you for allowance?"

"My parents are going to cosign my lease."

"Next week is my great-great-great-great grandmother's hundredth birthday!"

"You were *alive* when Kennedy got shot? Wow!"

Have you thought of roller-skating?

Ice-skating's fun, too.

Forget about your biological clock.

Sign up for swing dance lessons.

"What is youth except a man or woman
before it is ready or fit to be seen?"
—Evelyn Waugh

Take an improv class.

Have an ice-cream cone . . .

and make sure you ask for rainbow sprinkles.

"One of the signs of passing youth is the birth of a sense of fellowship with other human beings as we take our place among them."
—Virginia Woolf

Have a pizza . . .

with everything on it.

Wear your ponytail high so it bounces.

Treat yourself to expensive underwear.

"The excitement of learning separates
youth from old age. As long as you're
learning you're not old."
—Rosalyn S. Yalow

Learn a new language.

Fly a kite.

Volunteer for a political campaign.

March on Washington.

For awhile, taking estrogen after menopause
was supposed to be the answer to everything.
Then they said no, it was dangerous. But now
they're starting to think it may be the answer
to everything again.

"Begin at once to live, and count each
day as a separate life."
—Seneca

At least there are a lot more geriatricians than there used to be.

And some of them may have some good ideas about getting younger. After all, they're doctors!

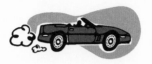

Purge These from
Your Vocabulary!

Social security

Girdle

Phonograph

Butterfield 8-3363

Dentures

Elderhostel

Leiderhosen

Cataract

Bone density

Burma

Burma-Shave

Daddy-O

Fondue party

Golden Oldies

aeroplane

velocipede

Cold War

Twenty-three skidoo

Senior discount

Senior moment

No thanks. I'm lactose-intolerant.

Whoa! Slow down!

We didn't have that when I was your age.

What's a video game?

Vitamin E plus exercise appears to help
improve lung function.

And to reduce blood sugar and
blood pressure levels.

And to reduce free radicals, even though no
one can ever remember what they are.

How 'bout that Astroglide!

"Youth is not a time of life; it is a
state of mind; it is not a matter of rosy cheeks,
red lips, and supple knees; it is a matter
of the will, a quality of imagination,
a vigor of the emotions; it is the freshness
of the deep springs of life."
—Samuel Ullman

OK, some creams that claim to get rid of wrinkles just "plump up" the skin instead of actually eliminating wrinkles. So what? You still can't see the wrinkles.

Try street hockey.

Think how much older your parents were when they were your age!

Some tortoises live to be one hundred.
Just figure out what they do, and copy it.

"Let us so live life that when we come to die
even the undertaker will be sorry."
—Mark Twain

Never refer to soap operas as "my stories."

Did you know that some people
can lower their blood pressure just by
imagining that it's going down?

Either have your varicose veins
removed, or stop caring about them.

And stop comparing symptoms
with your friends.

"Youth is, after all, just a moment,
but it is the moment, the spark, that
you always carry in your heart."
—Raisa Gorbachev

Stick to your own sleep patterns,
even if you go to bed at 4:00 a.m. and
sleep until 4:00 p.m.

(If your boss has trouble accepting
this idea, we'll write you a note.)

Become a child's mentor.

"Even though our bodies may age,
if we maintain an active, positive attitude,
our hearts and minds will remain 'youthful'
as long as we live."
—Daisaku Ikeda

It's not cool for you to dress like a teenager, but you can wear super-trendy sunglasses if you want.

Similarly, your handbag is allowed to be "of the moment."

"As I approve of a youth that has something of the old man in him, so I am no less pleased with the old man that has something of the youth. He that follows this rule may be old in body, but can never be so in mind."
—Marcus Tullius Cicero

Be even more careful about poison ivy as the years go by. The more often you're exposed to it, the worse its effect will be.

When you feel like taking a nap, take a walk instead.

(Then come home and take a nap.)

Go on all the scary rides at the amusement
park, unless you have a pacemaker.

"Too many people grow up. That's the real
trouble with the world, too many people grow
up. They forget. They don't remember what
it's like to be twelve years old. They patronize,
they treat children as inferiors."
—Walt Disney

Insist that the different foods on
your plate must not touch.

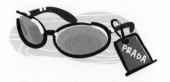

Somehow These People Have Always Been the Same Age!

Helen Mirren

Jack Nicholson

Steve Martin

Blythe Danner

Jimmy Carter

Maggie Smith

Judi Dench

Barbara Bush

Tina Turner

Suzanne Somers

Susan Sarandon

Diane Sawyer

Bill Cosby

Bill Clinton

Hillary Clinton

Cher

Mickey and Minnie Mouse

Candice Bergen

Dr. Dre

Dr. Joyce Brothers

Meredith Vieira

Ringo

Sam Waterston

Lisa Kudrow

Einstein (if he were still alive)

George Washington

Santa Claus

Give yourself nice presents on your birthdays, so you'll have something to look forward to.

Take a Shakespeare course. He must've said something wise about aging or maturity or something.

Take advantage of the gadgets that will make life easier, like jar openers and phones with bigger buttons. Why stress yourself out pretending you don't need them?

"The young do not know
enough to be prudent, and therefore they
attempt the impossible, and achieve it,
generation after generation."
—Pearl S. Buck

An egg yolk mask will tighten your skin.

A recent study suggests that even mild
exercise can reverse arterial damage.

Mnemonic devices really help when
you want to remember a list.

And if that doesn't work, you can
always write it down.

And if you lose your pencil, they make
teeny-tiny tape recorders these days.

There's another good technique for
remembering things, but we forget.

Did you really need to remember
that stupid list anyway?

"It is easy for us to criticize the prejudices of
our grandfathers, from which our fathers freed
themselves. It is more difficult to distance
ourselves from our own views, so that we can
dispassionately search for prejudices among
the beliefs and values we hold."
—Peter Singer

"Constantly choose rather to want
less, than to have more."
—Thomas à Kempis

A nice spiral notebook (wide-ruled) might make you feel like a sophomore this fall.

Nobody's making you celebrate your fiftieth birthday.

But if you do feel like throwing a party, you'll get lots of gifts.

Not to mention attention.

"I plan on living forever. So far, so good."
—Anonymous

A shower will make you feel at least
two months younger.

And a haircut—six minutes younger.

Might you feel younger by using
last year's calendar?

Having a much older spouse can
make you feel young . . .

So can having a much younger spouse!

Whistle a happy tune.

Whittling wood can be very satisfying. Don't laugh: It really can. Unfortunately, though, it doesn't do much for your staying young.

"I am in shape. Round is a shape."
—Anonymous

We don't know about you, but
having a clean desk makes us feel as if
we have a fresh start in life.

The hell with it. Life's too short
to put papers in piles.

Tuck your shirt in.

There's always "young at heart."

Acupuncture is supposed to be a savior.

The ice cream truck is here!
The ice cream truck is here!

A glass of wine every night won't kill you.

"I must take issue with the term 'a mere child,'
for it has been my invariable experience that
the company of a mere child is infinitely
preferable to that of a mere adult."
—Fran Lebowitz

You must have heard this before, but anyway:
Take the stairs instead of the elevator.

Substitute yogurt for sour cream.

Sometimes changing your hair part to the other side can do wonders.

A painless facelift? For no money?
It's called Photoshop.

Crossing the International Date Line
(west to east) will bring back a day.

If you can just figure out how to travel faster
than the speed of light, you can go back in
time—and then there's no end to how young
you can become . . .

Reinvent yourself.

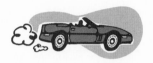

Jobs That Keep People Alive to One Hundred

Broadway playwright, producer, and director—George Abbott

TV Producer—Hal Roach

Baseball Player—Ted Radcliffe

Philanthropy—Brooke Astor

Politics—Alfred M. Landon, George Kennan,
Strom Thurmond

Author—Phyllis A. Whitney,
Kathleen Hale

Artist—Grandma Moses

Songwriter—Irving Berlin

General—James van Fleet

Mother of queen—Elizabeth,
Queen Mother

Mother of president—Rose Kennedy

Entertainer—Bob Hope, George Burns

Philosopher—Hans-Georg Gadamer

Ventriloquist—Señor Wences

Madame Chiang Kai-shek—
Soong Mei-Ling

Prosecutor at Nuremburg trials—
Hartley Shawcross

Actor who played Homer Bedloe on
Petticoat Junction—Charles Lane

Accidental synthesizer of LSD—
Albert Hofmann

Designer of the Sopwith Camel in
World War I—Thomas Sopwith

"Some people are making such thorough preparation for rainy days that they aren't enjoying today's sunshine."
—William Feather

Arm-toning exercises seem to work faster than ab-toners.

Watch fifteen minutes of MTV every day.

Dance studios now teach hip-hop the way
they used to teach the Hustle.

"There are only two ways to live your life.
One is as though nothing is a miracle. The
other is as though everything is a miracle."
—Albert Einstein

Yoga/mountain bike-type clothes
look good on any age.

(Plus, the pants are usually pretty stretchy.)

"A great many people think they
are thinking when they are merely
rearranging their prejudices."
—William James

If you don't have time for a full-blown nap, lie
on your back for ten minutes with
a pillow under your knees.

Have twins late in life, and all of a
sudden you'll appreciate how young you
were just nine short months ago.

Actually, having one baby early in life
will teach you the same lesson.

So will getting a kitten.

"You're never too old to become younger."
—Mae West

No matter how old you are, you're much, much younger than the Galapagos tortoises.

No matter how old you feel, you feel much, much younger than a woman your age would have felt in the eighteenth century.

No matter how old you look, you look much, much younger than . . . uh . . . those same Galapagos tortoises.

Older people are always complaining that young people throw things away instead of saving them or reusing them . . . so throw away lots of things instead of reusing them.

Did you ever consider taking in a foster child?

A Vespa might make you feel young . . .

but you'll look like a fool.

That goes double for a tricycle.

You could always trade in your
classical CDs for Raffi.

"If you aren't living on the edge,
then you are taking up too much space."
—Anonymous

Mashed banana is a wonderful moisturizer
for your skin and hair.

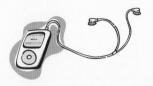

On the Other Hand:
Great Things About the Age
You Are Now

You can go to a party without having to worry about meeting Mr. Perfect.

You don't care who gets the last brownie in the pan.

Wrinkles are less embarrassing than zits.

You've slept in your last tent.

And turned in your last book report.

You don't have to ask the teacher for permission to go to the bathroom.

And you don't need a permission
slip to go on a trip.

You finally know what kind of
pillow works best for you.

You don't mind vaccines (and you don't
have to get many anymore).

You always have things like paper clips,
stamps, and extra toothbrushes.

No more scrounging for change—you have plenty of actual paper money now.

You're less likely to accidentally throw away your retainer when you dump your lunch tray.

No one cares whether you're wearing glasses.

You get to meet a lot of doctors.

You don't have to swim in cold
water if you don't want to.

And your friends don't splash you in the
swimming pool anymore.

Your sore knees give you compassion
for your fellow human beings.

You don't have to stay up late on
New Year's Eve.

The latest cataract surgery can give
you perfect vision.

You're safe even if they reinstate the draft.

People would actually prefer that you wear a
one-piece bathing suit with a skirt.

You're not scared of monsters
under your bed.

Athlete's foot is no longer a risk.

You've lived long enough to see
invisible stick deodorant.

A dab of olive oil will soften your lips.

Apply honey to your face and neck,
leave on for fifteen minutes, and voilà—
blemishes will (sort of) disappear.

"What would you attempt to do
if you knew you would not fail?"
—Robert Schuller

Cucumber slices soothe tired eyes.

And they also scare little children,
if that happens to be your goal.

Paddle your own canoe.

Pump your own gas.

Do your own taxes . . . no, wait, don't.

"Little people with little minds
and little imagination jog through life
in little ruts, smugly resisting all changes
which would jar their little worlds."
—Marie Fraser

Eat your dessert first.

Refuse to eat your vegetables.

Complain about your bedtime.

Push yourself harder when
you're feeling sluggish.

Cut yourself some slack when
you're feeling stressed.

"If you think nobody cares if you are alive,
try missing a couple of car payments."
—Earl Wilson

Drink a quart of milk a day.

(Or eat a gallon of ice cream.)

(Or pop some of those
delicious Viactiv caramels.)

Remember what you wanted to be when you grew up? There's still time!

"If you step on a crack, you'll break your mother's back." Live by this.

Get your car detailed.

Life's too short to make your
own wrapping paper.

Get a pedicure even if no one can
see it under your shoes.

You can get hand peels now, though
they're kind of pointless.

If, for some reason, you think it makes you look cool and youthful to ride a motorcycle, please wear a helmet.

"Show me a thoroughly satisfied man, and I will show you a failure."
—Thomas A. Edison

Although fasting isn't actually healthy, it makes you feel all light and floaty and pure.

Remind yourself to blink when
you're sitting at a computer. It will keep
your eyes from getting dry.

Put on your bathrobe, curl up in
front of a good movie, and dig into a
bowl of macaroni and cheese.

Only wear bright-red lipstick if you want to
add twenty years to your appearance.

When you're in the middle of a crisis, keep saying "I can handle this" to yourself.

One way to seem younger: Shriek "THAT'S MINE!" whenever someone touches anything of yours.

But lying down in the middle of the road and kicking is going too far.

Decorate a Christmas tree with a child.

Decorate with the help of a child, that is.
(We are the last people in the world
to endorse child ornaments.)

Make gingerbread cookies.

Wear sneakers in wacky color combinations.

Clutching a stuffed animal to your bosom
during a meeting at work is going too far . . .

So is snickering whenever someone
says the word "bosom."

So is bringing your lunch to work
in a Flintstones lunchbox.

But writing notes to the person sitting
next to you at the meeting is not.

Or doodling.

Write with a crayon.

"Twenty years from now you will
be more disappointed by the things
you didn't do than by the ones you did.
So throw off the bowlines. Sail away
from the safe harbor. Catch the trade
winds in your sails. Explore. Dream."
—Mark Twain.

Collect butterflies.

Play twenty questions.

Take an improv class.

Dance to a different drummer . . .

or at least take up the drums.

How long has it been since you did the limbo?

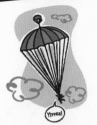

You Are How Young?

You are as young as you feel.

You are as young as the eyesight
of those around you.

You are as young as the oldness
of your mirror.

You are as young as the gullibility
of those you lie to.

You are as young as the person controlling
the lighting wants you to be.

You are as young as how long ago you
had your last appointment with the
physical therapist.

You are as young as the density of your bones.

You are as young as the number of inches you need to hold your book from your face when you're reading.

You are as young as the number of minutes it takes you to remember where you left your reading glasses.

You are as young as the amount you spend on skin care.

"If you want to be miserable, think about
yourself, about what you want, what you like,
what respect people ought to pay you and
what people think of you."
—Charles Kingsley

Start a scrapbook.

Sort your M&M's into colors
and throw away the greens.

Stir the ice cream in your
bowl until it's mushy.

Decide who's right by the
"rock, paper, scissors" method.

And if that's too mature-sounding, go for
"eenie, meenie, minie, moe."

When your boss criticizes you, shout "I know
you are, but what am I?"

Every day, pick a different friend to be mad at because she's "so stuck up."

And tell all your other friends not to speak to her either.

You should really look into having LASIK.

And they're talking about cataract surgery that can fix nearsightedness and farsightedness forever. Look into that, too!

Dunk your Oreos.

Did you know that speech lessons can help
make your voice warmer?

Be grateful for all the labor-saving
devices in modern life.

(In fact, be grateful, period.)

Take a walk through the supermarket
just to check out all the great new
foods they sell these days.

Ditto for the new products
in office-supply stores.

And hardware stores.

A trampoline is fun at any age.

And why don't you rent one of those inflatable "bounce castles" for your next party?

Or play musical chairs?

And bowling is always a nice party activity.

When you go out with a group of friends, make them walk in a line.

Choose the best behaved to be line leader.

And remember: buddy system!

Take a fall leaf-collecting walk.

Don't wear so much makeup that people
don't recognize you without it.

Make a lanyard out of gimp.

Play tag.

Refer to your parka as your "snowsuit jacket."

Make Valentine Day cards out of
construction paper and doilies and give
one to every person in your office.

Ask for toys for Christmas.

Fight with your brother and sister.

When trying to decide who should
have the last piece of pie, try the "one potato,
two potato" system.

Listen to a CD, talk on the phone, and watch
television at the same time.

"I want nothing to do with natural foods. At
my age I need all the preservatives I can get."
—George Burns

Have an argument with your mother about
what you're going to wear.

And always dress in a way that she says,
"You're going out in that?!"

Blast the music! To the max!

"Never give in, never give in, never;
never . . . in nothing, great or small,
large or petty . . . never give in except to
convictions of honor and good sense."
—Winston Churchill

Never clean your room.

Take hour-long showers.

And hog the bathroom generally.

Roll your eyes whenever your
mother or father speak to you.

"The best time to plant a tree is twenty
years ago. The second best time
to plant a tree is today."
—African Proverb

At your next bridge party, propose
a game of Go Fish instead.

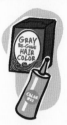

The Do's, Don'ts, and Do Nots of College Reunions

Don't worry. After the first five minutes of shock, everyone you know will look the same age as when you first met them.

Believe people when they say, "Everyone else has changed so much . . . except you!"

This is the time to splurge on the perfect pair of black pants.

This is not the time to learn Beer Pong.

Resist visiting your old dorm room. The current inhabitants will not appreciate it . . . and besides, what are those babies doing in a college dorm?

Practice the art of invisible name-tag-checking.

Don't bring your spouse if she or he
didn't go to college with you. You'll have
a lot more fun that way.

Make sure to attend the talent show!

(But don't be in it unless you
have a genuine talent.)

Some of the people you didn't know in
college will turn out to be even more
interesting than the ones you did know.

Say "you haven't changed!" to everyone,
even those you don't recognize.

Bring business cards.

Don't stay overnight in the dorms.

Be prepared for the food being worse
than you remembered.

Don't bring up that time you accused your
roommate of breaking your hair dryer.

Or the time you told her that she
left the bathroom a mess.

A lot of beautiful young actresses
swear by a macrobiotic diet.

(Then again, most of them smoke.)

When all else fails, get down on your knees
and pray to become younger.

Have pancakes for dinner sometimes.

Practice the things that matter, like skipping a stone five times.

And whistling through your teeth.

"You are remembered for the rules you break."
—Douglas MacArthur

Invite your friends over for a good
old-fashioned taffy pull.

(Then hire a cleaning service to get the taffy
out of your living-room rug.)

Get scuba-certified.

It doesn't matter about your hammertoes.
Go barefoot whenever you feel like it.

"It is an illusion that youth is happy, an
illusion of those who have lost it."
—W. Somerset Maugham

Remember that some aspects of childhood
are overrated—like piñatas.

And hopscotch.

And playing the triangle.

"Age is opportunity no less than youth itself, though in another dress, and as the evening twilight fades away, the sky is filled with stars, invisible by day."
—Henry Wadsworth Longfellow

Every day, give yourself a pat on the back for something you've done right.

Try a new recipe every week.

(And if you don't cook, order something you've never tasted at a restaurant.)

Make sure your hairdo can withstand sudden rain showers.

"A positive attitude may not solve
all your problems, but it will annoy enough
people to make it worth the effort."
—Herm Albright

In a rut? Climb out of it.

Spinning until you fall over is
cheaper than champagne.

At least people can't check how
old you are by looking in your mouth,
the way they do with horses.

Haven't you always wanted a
hammock in your living room?

Get over yourself!